Reflective Rhymes for
PATIENT CARE

Thought provoking pocket prose for health professionals

by Tammie Bullard

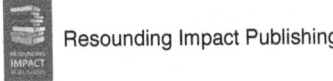
Resounding Impact Publishing

Copyright © 2020 Tammie Bullard

All rights reserved.

This publication or any part thereof may not be reproduced, distributed, transmitted or stored in a retrieval system in any form or by any means. This includes photocopying, recording, screen capturing or other electronic or mechanical methods, without prior written permission, except in the case of brief quotations when embodied in critical reviews and certain other non-commercial uses permitted by copyright law. For permission requests contact the author at www.gbuparamedic.com.

Reflective Rhymes for Patient Care

Artwork by Yukimura
Published by Resounding Impact Publishing

ISBN 978-0-6488808-9-9

*"Reflection is one of the most underused
yet powerful tools for success."*

Richard Carlson

Using Reflective Rhymes

The role that you play in healthcare, with every interaction, can make or break any patient's perception of an entire industry.

While it can become draining over months, years and decades, it doesn't have to negatively affect the way you, or they, feel when it's time to go home.

If finishing every shift, free from regret and filled with satisfaction is the secret to career longevity, then regular reflection may be the key to achieving that goal easily and often.

Reflective practice is not difficult, but building it into a regular routine can be. This book is designed to simplify that task.

- Select a topic for each week of the year or pick one at random when it suits.

- Read the rhyming paragraph several times and see which thoughts spring to mind.

- Make notes on where you're at right now and where you'd like to be in each section.

- Think about the rhyme while you work and whether you'd like to make changes.

- Re-visit and re-assess next time around to stay on track with your patient care approach.

Trainers, educators and facilitators can present each topic for group discussion and encourage reflection as a healthy habit.

Preceptors and mentors can use the rhymes as conversation starters, or to address behaviours and best practice issues whenever they arise.

With each reflection focusing on connection, team culture, communication, safety, public perception and respect for patients, peers and your profession, one per week will be plenty.

Reading them all at once is simply too much to digest and is likely to diminish their value.

Whichever way you choose to use this book in continued professional development, enjoy the process.

I hope that it proves useful in keeping every aspect of practice at the good end of the scale.

Thank you for having the dedication that motivates you to read, reflect and react with a desire to make a difference.

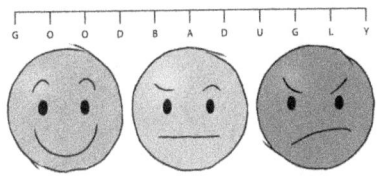

Growing the good, breaking the bad and undoing the ugly in patient care.

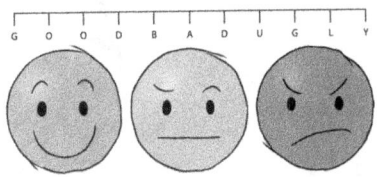

If our daily practice was secretly filmed

would it fill us with professional pride?

Or would watching it online and on TV

leave us shocked and dissatisfied?

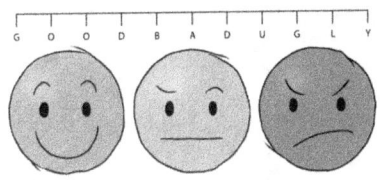

When we were students starting out

and saw behaviours that we respected,

did we adopt them fully for ourselves

and maintain them as much as we expected?

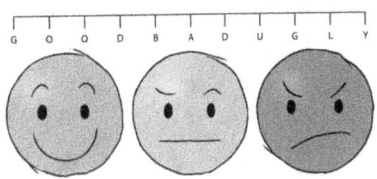

If we had been one of our patients

during our latest shift on call,

would it feel that we'd had concerns addressed

or had even been heard at all?

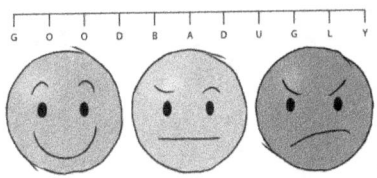

Are healthcare negatives continually discussed

with no focus on means for improvement?

Or does industry chatter encourage action,

towards positive change as a movement?

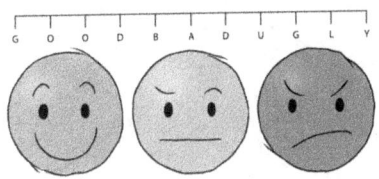

As new recruits, do we do our best

to learn from others every single day?

Or waste time learning swagger and bluff,

desperate to hide "newbie" status away?

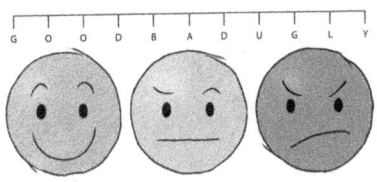

In coffee shops and restaurants,

when we gather as a uniformed collection,

does language, conversation and behaviour

ruin our profession's public perception?

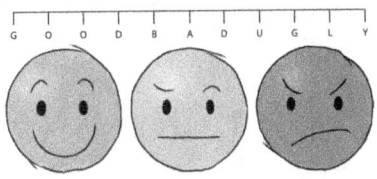

Is our documentation consistent,

no matter the time of day or night?

Would it stand up in court as true reflection

of everything we aimed to do right?

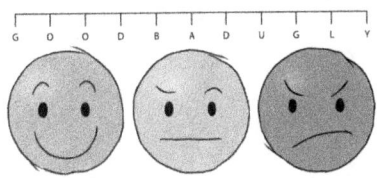

Are we comfortable saying "I don't know"

when conversing with patients and peers?

Or do we cover up gaps in knowledge

and bluff answers, just to hide our fears?

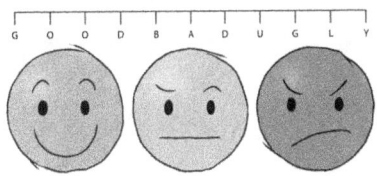

Where's the benefit to patients, or ourselves

if judgement makes us cold and uncaring?

Is harsh interaction more harmful to them

or our conscience that we end up despairing?

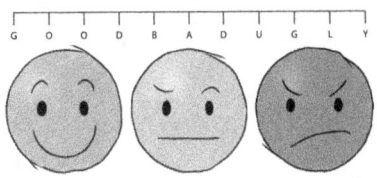

Do aseptic techniques

meet the standards they should?

Or could we make some improvement

to move from bad through to good?

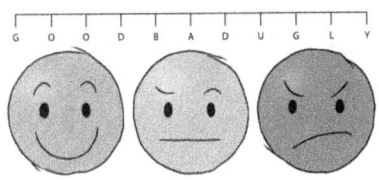

If we think of a time as a patient ourselves

when snubbed, dismissed or mistreated,

do we deliver care that outshines those ways,

or could our own patients feel just as cheated?

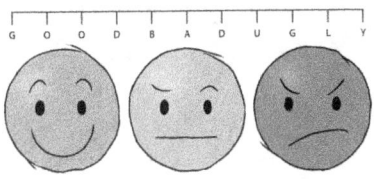

Do colleagues represent a united front

through the jobs and experiences they share?

Or undermine each other in front of patients,

until confidence is in complete disrepair?

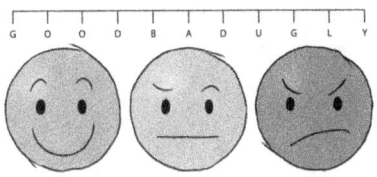

In leadership roles are we doing our best

so that staff feel just as well treated,

as the patients we expect them to care for?

Or would we hate our behaviours repeated?

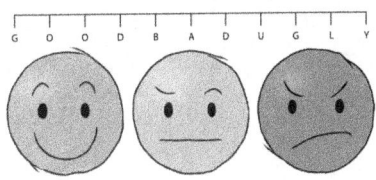

Do we wipe down equipment after every use

from shelves, trolleys and around the bed?

Are our daily standards really good enough,

for when a loved one is the patient instead?

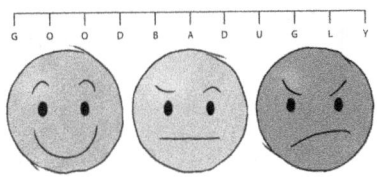

Should it make any difference if patients

are strangers or people we know?

Is it easier to always just deliver our best

so that professionalism is consistently on show?

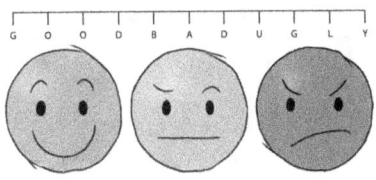

Are we supportive of each other,

with honest feedback, but still kind?

Or are we so competitive across the board

that we refuse to keep an open mind?

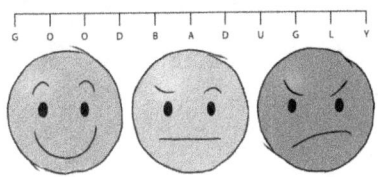

Reflecting on our most rewarding jobs

and what makes those memories so fond,

is it our skills, patients, the situation itself,

or that we went above and beyond?

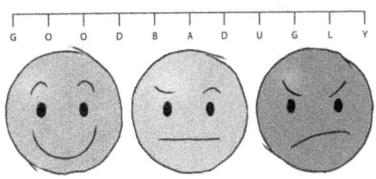

If aggressive "eat our young" culture

is still ingrained with no sign of improving,

are enough brave souls challenging its power

by rejecting, reducing and removing?

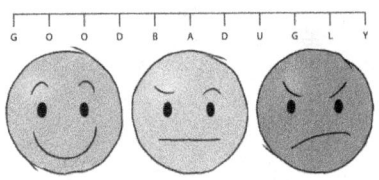

Does working on holidays and missing home

cause resentment towards those in our care?

Or do we appreciate that while we signed up,

few patients made a choice to be there.

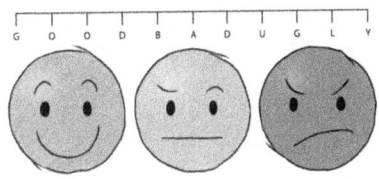

No matter how intelligent

each healthcare provider may be,

are we smart enough to cherish the value

in saying "I don't know" and "sorry?"

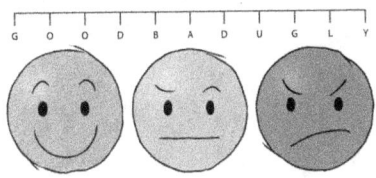

If we started over, fresh again

In our health professional careers,

which positive actions would we take

against bad habits cultivated over years?

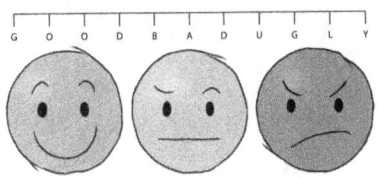

While we calm and soothe and reassure

our patients so they feel validated,

do we afford ourselves similar compassion,

or hide stress behind smokescreens created?

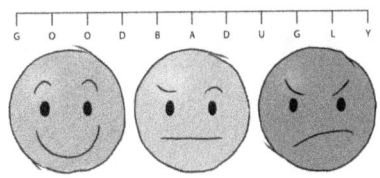

Do our reputations speak for themselves

with humility featuring high in the story?

Or is constant self-promotion required

to satisfy a need for glory?

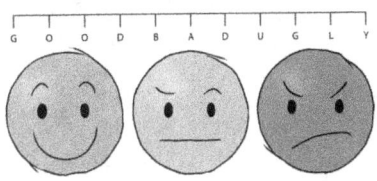

Do we go home after each shift,

sleeping soundly and free from regret?

Or feel disappointed that we gave much less

than we'd hope our loved ones would get?

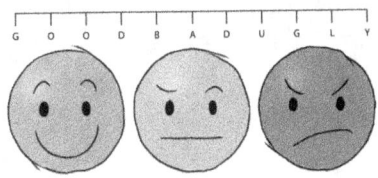

Are we kind and forgiving to ourselves,

so that we always carry enough,

to share with colleagues and patients

who may also be doing it tough?

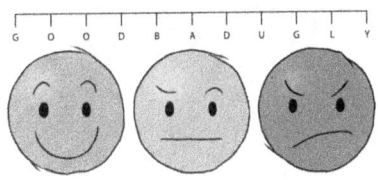

Is safety with sharps around colleagues given just as much thought and attention, as patients receive from our efforts towards needle stick injury prevention?

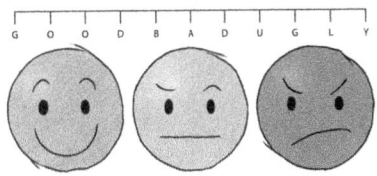

Are regular and repeat patients provided

the same standard of care and respect,

that we'd hope a loved one caught in that cycle

would receive and could grow to expect?

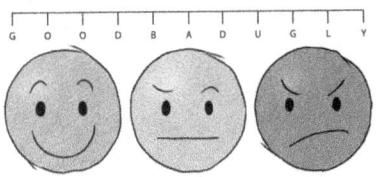

Are we careful when speaking, no matter

how conscious or altered patients are?

Or are we so comfortable in this setting

that they hear conversation going too far?

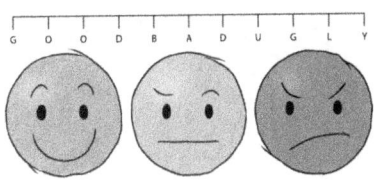

While there may be specific tips and tricks

that we're individually passionate about,

why force others to do it exactly our way

or risk having us call them out?

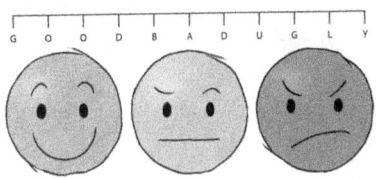

Is cutting a patient's clothing

only actioned as a last resort,

in case they can't afford replacements,

or do we grab the shears without thought?

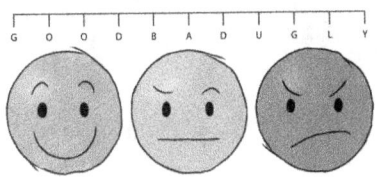

In precepting students and interns,

do we demonstrate our absolute best,

so they develop a habit of outstanding care

for when their own skills are put to the test?

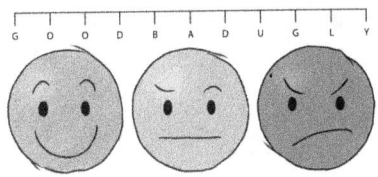

If effective communication and trust

are based on body language and tone,

do we focus enough attention on these

or rely on words and skills alone?

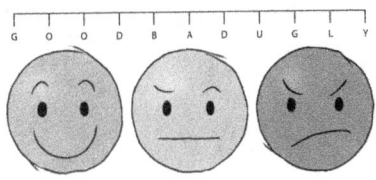

How do we respond to our colleagues

when they mention a tough case or shift?

Do we jump in, too fast, with opinion,

or listen fully, giving silence as a gift?

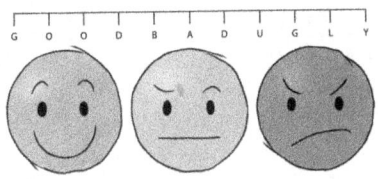

When watching a practitioner we admire,

which qualities do they seem to possess

that make us notice them amongst the crowd,

and are our standards just as high, or less?

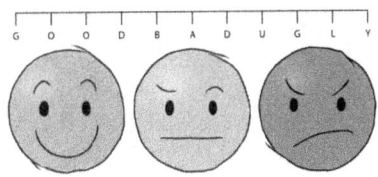

Burnt out, over it, compassion fatigue,

it's vital that we fend off this feeling.

Time for a break or change of scene

before hitting the proverbial ceiling?

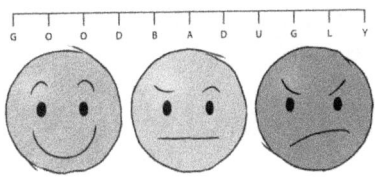

Are skills updated and practiced enough

on an individual self-driven basis?

Or only refreshed when they need to be used

in pressurised, high acuity cases?

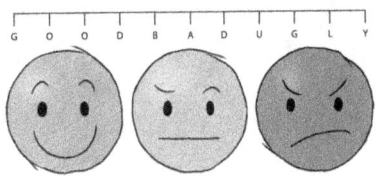

Does human connection suffer,

while we write up full documentation?

Could we interact with patients just a little more

for reassurance and validation?

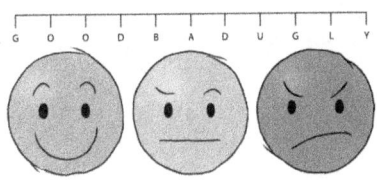

When we're forced to speak up for safety

to other health professionals and peers,

do we push aside confrontational dread

or say nothing rather than face our fears?

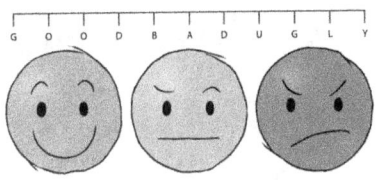

Do we speak just as kindly to ourselves

as we do to the patients we attend?

Could comments online, in person, in thought

be less harsh and perhaps more like a friend?

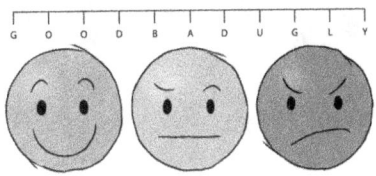

Words and actions are always remembered

by families when we deliver sad news.

Do we consistently give this the attention

that we'd hope for in those loved ones' shoes?

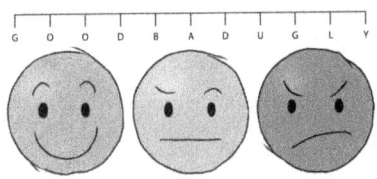

Do we choose IV cannula for its purpose,

or dependent on perceived behaviour?

Are large bores ever used in vengeance

on those patients we do not favour?

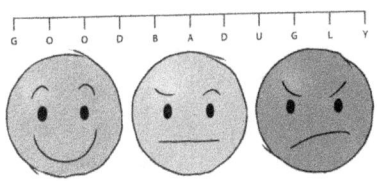

Do comments on lifestyle or appearance

feature heavily in our patient care?

Or do we keep those opinions private

with no need or entitlement to share?

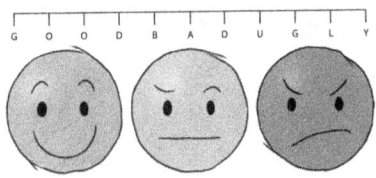

Is handover and discussion about patients

overheard by many others nearby?

Or carefully managed to take great care

that confidentiality remains high?

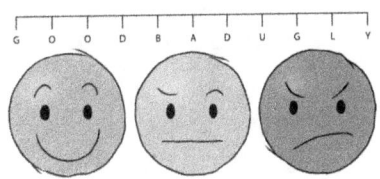

How much do we speak, and really connect

with the patients to whom we attend?

Are they active participants in proceedings,

or awkward observers, from start to end?

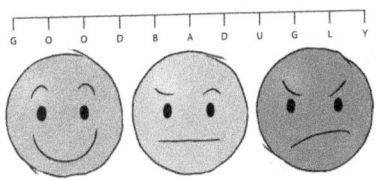

Does appreciation of support staff roles

shine through with respect and understanding?

Or are they treated with lesser importance,

with attitudes dismissive and demanding?

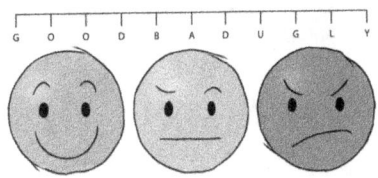

Is continued professional development

just a cross that we have to bear?

Or do we thrive on improving practice,

skills, knowledge and patient care?

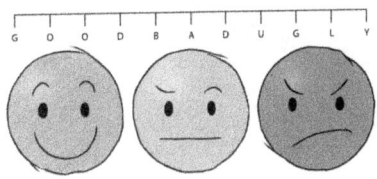

Is our profession based social media

for camaraderie, support and education?

Or has it simply become a place to vent,

laced with vitriol in every conversation?

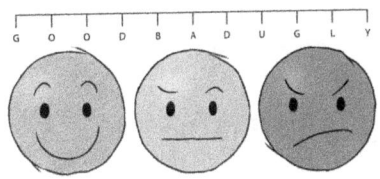

Do interactions with other professions

build bridges across the divide,

or dismiss them through lack of understanding

of their roles and the service they provide?

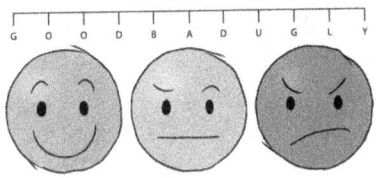

Though we may be on shift missing loved ones,

are we delivering the type of kindness and care,

that whether deemed worthy of our time or not

leaves no resentment or judgement in the air?

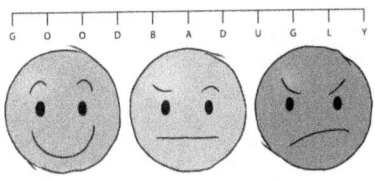

Through shifts spent in uniform,

do we consistently find

that work morals match personal,

or are they lagging behind?

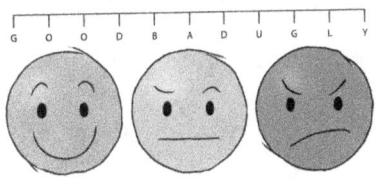

The humour we rely on may have great use

in defusing tense and stressful situations,

but are we using it for our own entertainment

or with kindness, for the benefit of patients?

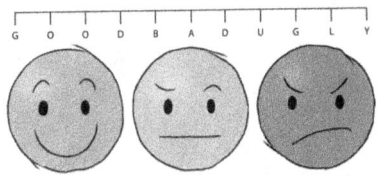

If given a chance to create the team

that treats us in the darkest of hours,

which qualities rank highly in their care,

and do they feature, right now, in ours?

I really appreciate your taking the time to reflect using this book. Feedback is incredibly valuable, so I'd love to hear any thoughts, good, bad or even ugly.

Reviews can be posted wherever
you obtained this copy or via:

Amazon
Facebook
Goodreads
Google Books
gbuparamedic.com/reviews

Free newsletter, articles and resources
available at www.gbuparamedic.com
and social platforms @gbuparamedic

Thank you for your tireless efforts in caring
for others through your dedicated role.

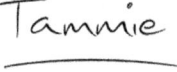

About The Author

Tammie Bullard is a writer, author and paramedic with a passion for professionalism and patient care.

An academic journey from undergraduate to postgrad qualifications in intensive care paramedicine, and a master's degree in critical care, ignited her interest and sparked a habit of writing.

Through emergency ambulance and teaching roles such as preceptor, trainer, clinical support paramedic, university lecturer and unit co-ordinator, she is intrigued by recurring cultural chatter around the question of what constitutes "good" patient care.

After publishing "The Good, The Bad & The Ugly Paramedic" in 2019, all manner of healthcare professionals have cited the benefits gained from its simple pain scale approach to reflective practice.

Written with every patient care provider in mind, this pocket guide is designed to keep us thinking, questioning and assessing. Ensuring that our own approaches meet the standards we'd want from each other, when our loved ones need it most.

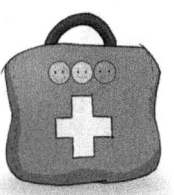

www.ingramcontent.com/pod-product-compliance
Lightning Source LLC
Chambersburg PA
CBHW050319010526
44107CB00055B/2303